MW00905529

HEALTHY HABITS

21 Evening Habits That Help You Lose Weight, Live Healthy & Sleep Well

by Linda Westwood

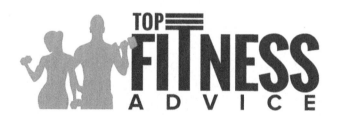

Copyright © 2017 By Linda Westwood
All rights reserved. No part of this book may be reproduced in any
form without permission in writing from the author. No part of this
publication may be reproduced or transmitted in any form or by any
means, mechanic, electronic, photocopying, recording, by any
storage or retrieval system, or transmitted by email without the
permission in writing from the author and publisher.
For information regarding permissions write to author at
Linda@TopFitnessAdvice.com.
Reviewers may quote brief passages in review.

Linda Westwood
TopFitnessAdvice.com

Table of Contents

Who is this book for?

Do you feel that your nighttime binges and cravings ruin your diet?

Are you struggling to stick to healthy habits and lose weight?

Are you one of those people who *know* what to do, but struggle to *actually do* it?

Then this book is for you!

I am going to share with you some of the MOST effective evening habits that you can add into your life to lose weight, feel great and sleep well!

I have given you a simple action plan at the end of each chapter so you can implement each habit very easily!

Also, you don't have to be overweight to benefit from these habits.

Yes, they help you lose weight, but they also help you live a healthy life, as well as sleep well at night!

What will this book teach you?

This book is not like others!

It doesn't just contain generic advice that we all already know, but actual evening habits that have been identified to INCREASE weight loss, IMPROVE sleep quality, and LEAD to a more healthy life!

Some of these habits are very simple and you can begin implementing them from tonight, and some are a little more difficult, in that you will need to practice them more!

I will also share with you why each of these habits work and are so effective – along with a simple action plan to help get you started and on your way to lasting success!

Introduction

A lot of people will tell you that getting a good fresh start to the day is the most important part of leading a happy, healthy life.

But the secret to getting that fresh start is building the right habits the night before.

The evening is your time to decompress and rejuvenate yourself. It is your time to strengthen your resolve and recharge your batteries so that tomorrow morning, you actually can wake up feeling fresh and ready to take on the day.

Your evening routine can make or break your weight loss plan. Even after spending the whole day staying strong and sticking to a healthy diet, it could all be undone by your midnight snacking in front of the television when you get home at night.

Snacking—especially when you're snacking on junk food right before you go to sleep—can pack on more calories than you even realize.

And once you fall asleep, your metabolism drops into low gear and ends up just storing most of those extra calories as fat.

So if you've been trying to lose weight but have found yourself stagnating and unable to burn those finicky pounds, it might be because your evening habits are holding you back (and holding the weight on).

Unfortunately, most diet plans and health advice focus on what you should be doing in the mornings and during the day. But after dinnertime, they've got little to no advice.

At most, they'll simply say, "don't snack after dinner" or "get a good night's sleep" as if just telling yourself to do it will actually make it happen.

Almost every healthy weight loss habit is easier said than done but that doesn't mean they are impossible. This book is here to give you real advice that you can really use.

It won't just tell you "don't snack after dinner", it will give you a solid action plan for *how* to undo that nasty post-dinner snacking habit. You'll get in depth details and step by step advice for eliminating the bad habits that are holding you back and cultivating the good habits that will help you finally shed that extra weight once and for all.

A healthy and rejuvenating end to the day is just as important as that fresh start. Speed up your weight loss by cutting out those weight gain causing habits and replace them with effective yet simple weight loss strategies.

We won't pretend it's easy but it *is* easier than you think, especially if you know exactly what you can do to accomplish it.

There are 21 healthy evening habits in this book. Each of them will help you lose weight faster. But if you really want to increase your chances of losing weight and keeping it off, don't overwhelm yourself by deciding to start doing all 21 habits at once.

Take them a step at a time. Give each habit the time it deserves to become fully incorporated into your daily routine.

If you give each habit time, it will actually become a full habit, meaning you won't have to constantly remind yourself to do it and you won't find yourself struggling to keep up with it.

You'll actually change the way you do things and finally get rid of those unhealthy habits that have been packing on pounds faster than you can burn them off.

So read through each step, learn why it works, and then read the action plan for how to actually incorporate it into your routine. In addition to individual tips for adopting each habit, you'll get a sample calendar for a 30-day challenge in the last chapter.

This calendar will help you adopt all 21 habits in a way that will help make sure you stick with them for the long term.

Each habit from this book will help you either cut more calories or burn more calories so the more habits you pack on, the more pounds you are going to see drop off!

Read This FIRST - 100% FREE BONUS

FOR A LIMITED TIME ONLY – Get Linda's best-selling book *"Quick & Easy Weight Loss: 97 Scientifically Proven Tips Even For Those With Busy Schedules!"* absolutely FREE!

Readers who have read this bonus book along with this book have seen the greatest changes in their weight loss both *FAST & EASILY* and have improved overall fitness levels – so it is *highly recommended* to get this bonus book.

Once again, as a big thank-you for downloading this book, I'd like to offer it to you *100% FREE for a LIMITED TIME ONLY!*

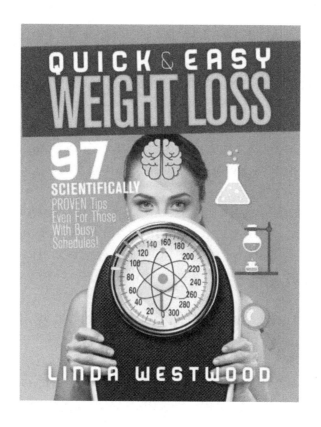

Get your free copy at:

TopFitnessAdvice.com/Bonus

Evening Habit #1 – Slow It Down!

One of the most important habits you can practice is eating slowly.

You need to take your time with food rather than just shoveling it down while you drive to work.

Eating slowly might not seem like it would change how many calories you eat, just how long it takes you to eat them. But it does actually help you reduce the number of calories and keep you feeling full between meals.

Multiple studies have been done which show that people who eat slowly also eat less.

In one study, the participants who ate slowly ate an average of 100 calories less than the participants who ate quickly.

In another study, participants were all given the same amount of ice cream. Some were told to eat it in 5 minutes and others were told to eat it in 30 minutes.

Those who spent 30 minutes eating the ice cream had a higher concentration of hormones in their stomach that caused them to feel fuller for longer.

This means that the physical signal (the hormones) to feel full will be stronger if you eat slowly so you feel full sooner and you keep feeling full longer.

So, if you make slow eating a habit, you'll eat fewer calories in one meal and avoid adding more calories between meals.

This habit alone can dramatically reduce the total number of calories you eat in a day, which will help you lose weight much more quickly.

Fast eating not only causes you to eat more total calories, it doesn't let your body produce enough of the hormone that makes you feel full.

Without that hormone, you could eat 1,000 calories and still feel hungry enough to eat a horse because the full feeling you should have just isn't there.

On the other hand, if you eat slowly, you could eat a 300-calorie meal and be so full that you feel as if you *did* just eat a horse.

Plus, that full feeling will last for hours after you've eaten so you're less likely to want to snack between meals.

The bottom line: eating *less* food can make you feel *more* satisfied if you eat it slowly.

But there are even more benefits to eating slowly than just eating less and feeling fuller. You also get more pleasure from your food.

When you eat slowly, you are giving yourself the time to savor and enjoy every single bite. You get the full experience of the food on your plate and the full range of flavors it has to offer.

Getting more pleasure out of your meal time is more important than you might think. Our brains have evolved to seek out pleasure and avoid pain.

In the case of food, our brains are seeking out the pleasure of eating and avoiding the pain of feeling hunger. So, when you don't take the time to enjoy your meal, your brain isn't getting the pleasure signal it's looking for which means it's going to keep looking for more food even though you've literally just eaten.

At the physiological level, feeling pleasure releases certain neurotransmitters and hormones in the body.

These neurotransmitters and hormones are what give you the physical sensations that come with pleasure: relaxed muscles, reduced pain, lower blood pressure, and the emotional and physical feeling of wellbeing.

This same pleasure process that is making you feel more relaxed is responsible for turning your metabolism. That means that simply taking the time to enjoy your meal can increase your metabolism.

If that's not enough to convince you, the hormones that make you feel stressed actually slow down your metabolism. So, eating quickly and feeling rushed while you eat can actually slow down your metabolism.

At the physical level, stress hormones are your body's way of knowing that it needs to start planning for a worst-case scenario. It slows down digestion and stores more of the calories as fat because it thinks it should prepare for a famine.

Your body can't tell the difference between stress about work and stress about not having enough food. So, when you feel stressed or guilty while eating, you are causing your body to store fat.

When you feel pleasure while eating, you are telling your body that everything is fine and there is no need to store any fat for later.

So, to sum it all up, eating slowly and enjoying your meal has three powerful weight loss effects in your body:

1. Decreased total calorie intake

2. Increased production of the hormone that makes you feel full

3. Increased metabolism

So, you eat less, you feel full for longer, and you burn the calories more quickly.

All of that happens just because you took your time to eat and enjoy food!

Action Plan

Now that you know why it's so important to eat slowly and enjoy your meal, it's time to learn how you can actually start doing it.

When you first start, it's going to be difficult to slow down your pace for the entire meal. You'll feel a little impatient and have a hard time resisting the impulse to just keep shoveling in bite after bite.

But you can and should do it.

Since you want to increase pleasure as well, it might not be good to time yourself for each bite. It could just end up stressing you out.

Instead, slow down by taking time to enjoy the food. Take one bite at a time. Put your fork or spoon down after you take the bite. Chew your food slowly and let it roll over your tongue.

Be aware and consciously think about the different flavors and textures that you are experiencing.

You can make a game out of it by trying to recognize every ingredient in the dish.

Is that a hint of rosemary you taste?

Maybe there's a dash of cinnamon.

Even if you made it yourself and already know every ingredient that is in it, try to actually recognize each ingredient that you added.

Once you have swallowed the bite, take a sip of water—or wine, whatever you are drinking with your meal. Then, pick your fork back up and take the next bite. Take the time to experience and enjoy that one, too.

If you still find that you're having a hard time slowing down, there are actually apps available for your smartphone that help you eat slowly. Many of them are free so try downloading one and using it to help you get into the habit of slow eating.

You might be thinking that eating slowly and enjoying your meal sounds great in theory but you just don't have the   time   to   do   it.

If that's the case, make time.

It's time to end the "working lunches", and wake up a little earlier to give yourself the time for a relaxing, enjoyable breakfast.

You have read all the benefits of eating slowly and eating with pleasure so you know that it's worth making room in your schedule to do it.

Evening Habit #2 – Stop Eating After Dinner

After-dinner snacking is the mortal enemy of any diet plan. It can undo all your efforts during the day to stick to your diet. It's not just the added calories but also the way you eat them and when you are eating them.

In almost every case, snacking after dinner happens while you are sitting in front of the TV and not actually paying any attention to the food you are eating.

You have just finished reading through the first evening habit of eating slowly so you already know why it's so important to pay attention to your food while you eat it.

You end up eating way more than you should and you hardly gain a fraction of the satisfaction you should be getting from it which means that your body doesn't have a chance to make the food-pleasure connection that you need in order to put cravings to rest.

Beyond that, it's also a lot of extra calories that you are taking on even though your dinner should have provided you with enough to get you through the rest of the night.

You eat all these extra calories and then, what?

You go to sleep—an activity that requires the bare minimum of calories. So you just took in a bunch of extra calories and then went on to do a low calorie activity.

Your body has no other choice but to store those extra calories as fat.

In one study, participants were told to stop after dinner snacking for two weeks. They didn't change anything else at all about their eating habits or exercise habits.

After two weeks, they lost 1 pound (just from cutting out evening snacks). But what is even more interesting about this study is the fact that after the two weeks, they were told to spend one week going back to their old routine of nighttime snacking.

In that one week, they *gained* an average of 1.3 pounds. The only change was the evening snacking and they gained back all the weight they lost plus a little extra.

This simple habit of cutting out after dinner snacks could cut about 250 calories from your daily total (depending on how many calories you tend to eat after dinner).

That translates to about ½ a pound per week lost, just because you said no to your usual snack.

If you combine this with first habit, you could be cutting out more than 500 calories from your daily total every single day.

Even if you make absolutely no other changes aside from these two things, that's already going to help you lose about 1 pound per week!

Action Plan

If you snack after dinner every night or almost every night, it's probably become a deeply engrained habit that will be hard to break but it's definitely worth the effort.

So, what's the most simple and effective strategy for cutting out after dinner snacks?

Just stop snacking after dinner!

If you've got any willpower, just fight the urge.

But if that strategy isn't working for you, get more creative with it: put up "closed" signs on the fridge or pantry after dinner to remind you that snack foods are off limits.

It sounds silly but having a big sign on the fridge when you go to open it makes it impossible to forget that you are not supposed to be getting any snacks.

If the urge to snack is starting to feel like more than you can bear, do something else.

Go for a walk (evening habit #11) or work on a craft. The need to feed will go down if you are keeping your mind and body actively involved in something else.

You'll learn more about this when you learn about evening habits #11 and #12.

One of the best ways to keep from snacking is to not have snacks!

Just don't buy them. Even if your kids throw a fit, they'll get over it eventually. Any food that can be eaten without any preparation (except for fruits and vegetables) should just be kept out of your kitchen. This might sound like a difficult adjustment to make but you'll learn more about later in this book. Evening habit #19 is all about snack-free shopping.

In fact, if post-meal snacks are a serious problem for you, many of the habits in this book will help you finally break the snacking routine and cut hundreds of calories from your daily total!

So, keep on reading to learn more about how you can avoid snacking, cut total calories, and boost your metabolism so that you can finally lose the weight that's been burdening you!

Evening Habit #3 – If You Eat, Don't Cheat

No matter how strong your will power is, there are going to be some days when you simply can't avoid having a snack to help you make it through to the next meal.

Sometimes, you just won't have the time to cook a full, balanced, healthy meal. Life can be hectic and you can't always devote as much time to your health as you would like to.

Luckily, there are some ways around this and there are habits you can build to make sure that even when you don't have time, you can still eat healthy and make sure you don't undo all the progress you have made.

From planning your meals to snacking properly, you'll be able to keep your calorie count in a reasonable range and continue to lose weight no matter how busy you are.

The trick is to choose healthy, low calorie snacks that are satisfying to munch on without loading you up with extra calories.

Your first line of defense, however, is making sure you have well-planned meals that are high in fiber and protein so that you can be sure you feel full between meals.

In the next section of this chapter (the action plan), you'll learn how to make a meal plan for the week that will fight cravings and keep your total number of calories low enough that you can shed the extra weight.

If you still have cravings between meals even though you've planned them so well, there are some healthy snacks that you can keep in the house that won't break the calorie bank.

These are all foods that, after digestion, have a very minimal caloric impact.

Some of these foods also have metabolism-boosting and appetite-controlling effects so they can help control your cravings and increase the rate at which you burn calories.

Of course, it's better not to snack at all because then your body will focus on burning the calories already stored as fat.

But, if you absolutely have to munch on something, choose a minimal calorie food so that you aren't adding too many new calories.

Here are a few low-calorie foods you can snack on:

- Carrots
- Broccoli
- Spinach
- Radishes
- Cucumbers
- Melons (cantaloupe, honeydew, etc.)
- Peaches
- Pineapple

- Strawberries
- Mangoes
- Tangerines
- Garlic
- Onion
- Cinnamon
- Flax seed
- Cayenne pepper
- Chili powder

You'll get a few other healthy snack ideas in chapter 19 when you learn about snack-free shopping.

At the end of the list, you got a few seasonings and some foods that you probably don't want to eat plain (like garlic or onion).

Combine these foods together to create tasty, low-calorie meals.

For example, slice up a mango and dust it with cayenne and chili powder.

It might sound strange but the spice of the cayenne and chili powder really complements the sweetness of the mango for an exciting flavor contrast.

Toss some spinach with flax seeds, strawberries, and tangerines for a salad that is flavorful enough to be delicious without any diet-busting salad dressing.

There are a lot of healthy options for snacking that won't add calories so there's no excuse for cheating on your diet just because your stomach is grumbling between meals.

Action Plan

As mentioned earlier, the best defense against between meal cravings is a well-designed meal plan and thorough preparation.

If your weeks tend to be really busy and you often come home feeling too tired to prepare and cook a balanced, diet-friendly meal, then you should start preparing in advance.

To do this, you'll need to make a menu for the entire week. This includes 3 meals for each day on every day of the week. Then, you'll write out your list of ingredients (including the exact amounts needed of each one) and go shopping.

Once you've got all your ingredients, you'll prepare all your meals for the week.

Then all you have to do is store them in the meal-sized portions in the freezer.

Throughout the week, you can come home, pull a meal out of the freezer and just reheat it for a completely balanced and satisfying meal without all the work.

Now, when you come home exhausted and hungry, you won't have to do any heavy cooking. You get to combine the convenience of processed, store-bought meals with the health and weight loss power of a fresh, home-cooked meal!

It's best to do this on the weekend when you have more time. On Saturday or Sunday, spend the morning and afternoon planning, shopping, and cooking.

Then, prepare to sit back and relax for the rest of the week!

As you plan your menu, make sure that you cover all your bases and come up with satisfying, healthy meals.

Here are some key things to consider as you plan:

1. The average person needs 25 to 30 grams of fiber daily. This means each meal should have about 10 grams of fiber.
   a. Whole grains, beans, legumes, and oatmeal are a few good options to meet your fiber requirements.

2. The average person needs about 50 grams of protein per day. So, each meal should have roughly 16 or 17 grams of protein in it.
   a. Beans, legumes, egg yolks, nuts, yogurt, seeds, fish, seafood, and poultry are all healthy sources of protein that won't hurt your blood pressure or cholesterol levels (in fact, they will help lower both of these things).

3. The average person needs to eat about 30 grams of fat every day. This means about 10 grams per meal.

a. As strange as it sounds, you do also need fat in your diet if you want to burn fat. Healthy fat (unsaturated fats) help fight high cholesterol and stabilize your blood glucose levels so that you don't get between meal cravings.
b. The key is to look for *unsaturated* fat. As you increase the amount of unsaturated fat, decrease the amount of saturated fats and Trans fats. Try to cut Trans fats out completely. Keep saturated fats down to around 3 to 5 grams.
c. Nuts, seeds, oils (olive, sesame, or coconut), fish, avocados, and olives are all great sources of unsaturated fats.

Each meal should contain something from each category. Make sure there are also at least one or two servings of fruits or vegetables in each meal.

Fruits are especially good to include in your breakfast because the fructose (sugar) will provide an immediate energy boost while the protein, fiber, and fat from the rest of your breakfast will provide sustained and stable energy throughout the day.

Your lunch should also have a couple servings of fruit as well to give you a quick boost while you wait for the protein, fiber, and fat to provide sustained energy.

Avoid fruits or other simple sugars at dinner though, because you don't want a sharp spike in your blood glucose levels keeping you awake when it's time to go to bed.

If you make sure that you have a wide variety of healthy whole foods throughout the day, you won't have to worry about counting calories or tediously tallying up all your vitamins and minerals.

The variety of different fruits, vegetables, grains, and proteins will help make sure that you are getting all the nutrients you need without packing on too many calories.

Focus on including a lot of different nutrient-dense foods and skip all the "low fat" and "diet" versions of foods.

In order to make a food low fat, manufacturers usually add a lot of extra sugar to make up for the loss in flavor. But sugar (*not* fat) is one of the leading causes of weight gain.

Diet foods often contain artificial and heavily processed ingredients (like hydrogenated fats and artificial sweeteners).

These artificial ingredients are things your body has no idea how to break down and use so, instead of digesting them, it simply stores them as fat until it can figure out what to do with them. Basically, "diet" soda and other "diet" foods are actually causing you to gain more weight.

Your best option is to stick to natural, whole foods—foods with ingredients that you can identify. If there's a long list of unpronounceable ingredients, put it back on the shelf and move on.

Once you have created your healthy menu for the week, gather all your ingredients and spend the afternoon cooking. When you cook in bulk and cook all at once, you'll spend less total time cooking than you would if you prepared each meal separately throughout the week.

Your breakfasts may be simple enough that you can just prepare them every morning instead of making them all at once and storing them. But your lunches and dinners probably need to be prepared in advance so that you can save time during the week without sacrificing your goal of losing weight or your health.

You can make your weekly cooking day a fun family activity. Teach your children the same healthy habits that you are trying to adopt so they grow up with the right attitudes and skills toward food to live long, healthy, happy lives.

If you are liking these tips so far, *you must* check out my 97 weight loss tips that are available to you right here!

If the link is still active, get it while you can, because I will be removing it soon (I can't keep giving away AWESOME secrets like these for free *forever*).

Evening Habit #4 – Cut This Out & Lose Weight FASTER Than Before!

Of all the meals of the day, your dinner should take the longest to digest. You want foods that are slow to break down so that your stomach is too busy digesting in the evening to feel cravings.

What this means is that you want a lot of protein and fat without as many simple carbohydrates.

Of all the kinds of foods out there, carbohydrates digest the fastest. This leads to sharp spikes in your blood glucose levels followed by equally sharp drops.

This is exactly what causes cravings—especially cravings for sweets.

When your body experiences sudden and fast drops in blood glucose, it begins to panic and look for more carbohydrates to quickly restore your glucose levels.

So try to cut out carbohydrates from your dinner.

At the very least, you need to cut out simple carbohydrates.

Simple carbohydrates are sugars, refined flours, and starchy foods (potatoes, sticky rice, etc.) A good way to identify and eliminate simple carbohydrates is to remember to avoid white foods: white bread, refined white sugar, potatoes, and so on.

Of course, there are some white foods that don't fit on this list (milk, cauliflower, etc) but in general, this is how you can safely avoid simple carbohydrates.

Complex carbohydrates are the ones that take more time for your body to digest like high fiber foods and vegetables. They still digest more quickly than proteins and fats but it's slow enough (and adds enough nutrition to your diet) that you don't need to avoid them.

The reason you want to cut down the carbohydrates at dinner is because you don't need the energy boost they offer when you're just going to be relaxing and then going to bed.

Instead, you want your dinner to be a meal that digests slowly and keeps your stomach busy all night so that you are less likely to run to the kitchen for a late-night snack before bed.

Action Plan

Make protein and fat the key parts of your dinner without going over your calorie budget by slightly decreasing the amount of protein and fat you eat for breakfast and lunch.

For example, to get your 50 grams of protein, eat 12 grams for breakfast, 13 grams for lunch, and 25 grams for dinner.

To get the 30 grams of fat, you can eat 5 grams at breakfast, 5 grams at lunch and 20 grams at dinner.

Between 25 grams of protein and 20 grams of fat, your dinner is going to easily keep you full through the night.

At the same time that you are increase the protein and fat, decrease the carbohydrates. You need 30 grams of fiber (which comes exclusively from complex carbohydrate foods).

To get this, eat 10 grams for breakfast, 15 grams for lunch and 5 grams at dinner.

The other benefit of making your breakfast and lunch high in complex carbohydrates while your dinner is high in protein and fat is that the carbohydrates give you a faster boost to your glucose levels (i.e. - your energy).

That means that during the day, when you need to have the most energy, your meals are giving you the perfect balance of fast-acting energy and stable, sustained energy.

Come dinner when it's time to relax and slow down, you'll have a slow-digesting meal that will help keep you from getting late night cravings and avoid those extra, after dinner snacks.

Avoid simple carbohydrates throughout the day, every day. The only sugar that you should be getting is the small amount that comes from fruits.

Cut out *all* foods that have added sugar. If you have a serious sweet tooth, this will be difficult at first. But trust me, after a few weeks of sticking to the no-added sugar rule, it will get easier and easier.

Soon, you'll be able to enjoy the natural sweetness of fruits and even start disliking excessively sugary foods.

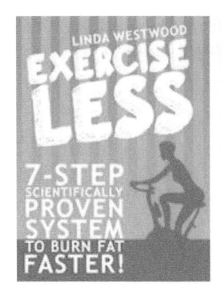
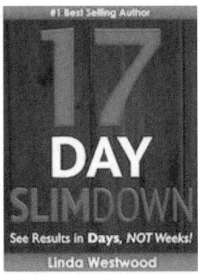
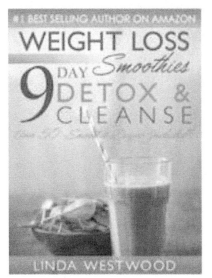
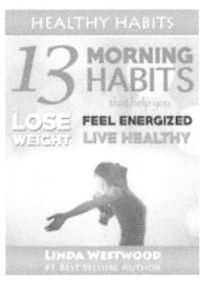

Check out Linda's books at:

TopFitnessAdvice.com/go/books

Evening Habit #5 – Make Sleep a Priority

Your first thought might be: how can sleep possibly help me lose weight?

You burn the *least* amount of calories while sleeping. Well, this chapter will explain the very important role that sleeps plays in weight loss and your overall health.

It won't take a lot of convincing to tell you that you need to get a good night's sleep every night.

You probably already know the difference between how you feel after a night of quality sleep in comparison to a night of too little sleep.

But it does more than just make you feel more alert and energized in the morning.

Here are some of the other reasons that sleep is so essential:

1. Lack of sleep causes cravings: when you wake up feeling tired and unenergetic, you usually reach for a big cup of coffee and a sugary treat to give you the boost you need.

   If you had gotten a good night sleep, you would wake up feeling naturally energized and alert. Instead of desperately going for a fast sugary boost, you could prepare and eat a healthy, balanced breakfast.

2. Lack of sleep slows metabolism: just as you lack energy in the morning after a bad night of restless sleep, so does your metabolism.

   Your digestive system is triggered by the same hormones that regulate your sleep cycle. The hormone that tells your brain to feel alert also tells your metabolism to rev up and start producing energy.

   Without enough sleep, you don't get these wake-up hormones (because your body literally doesn't want you to wake up yet) which means your metabolism doesn't get the signal to start working.

3. Sleep helps you avoid late night snacking: the logic is simple enough. If you are asleep, you can't eat (well, unless you are a sleep-eater).

   So instead of staying up until 3am surfing on the internet, get to bed early enough (at least 6 or 7 hours before you plan to wake up) to make sure that you get a full night of sleep and avoid the midnight munchies.

4. Sleep helps you burn fat: studies show that sleep helps your body burn fat. Two people who eat the exact same low calorie diet will not burn the same amount of fat if they don't get the same amount of sleep.

   For example, in one study, people ate the same number of calories but one group slept 8.5 hours per night while the other group slept just 5.5 hours per night.

By the end of the study, both groups had lost an average of 6.5 pounds. But when they measured where those pounds came from, the results were surprising.

For the group that slept 5.5 hours per night, only 25% of those pounds were from fat. For the group that got a full night of sleep, however, more than 50% of the pounds lost were fat.

5. Sleep helps you eat less calories: not only does it help you stop snacking late at night but it helps you naturally lower the number of calories you eat during the day.

Many studies have been done on this subject and they have found that people who get a full night of sleep eat an average of 700 fewer calories per day than people who don't get enough sleep.

That is a truly significant amount. 700 fewer calories per day could translate to up to 2 pounds of weight loss per week!

Action Plan

Now that you know how important sleep is and how it can help you with your weight loss and health goals, it's time to learn how you can make sure that you sleep better and get the sleep that you need.

The first step is to stop doing things that are hurting your ability to fall asleep and sleep well.

Here are some of the things that you need to stop doing:

1. **Stop looking at screens**: the backlight that comes out of your computer screen, phone screen, tablet screen, or television screen is a similar frequency as the light that comes from the sun.

   Because your body is programmed to respond to sunlight as a signal that it's time to be awake and alert, looking at screens (which emit light similar to sunlight) can damage your body's natural sleep and wake cycle.

   You don't have to give up technology altogether. But you do need to put it away and stop using it 4 hours before you plan to go to sleep.

2. **Stop eating before bed**: eating right before bed so that you have a bloated, full stomach will make it more difficult for you to fall asleep because your body is too busy digesting to fall into the relaxed mental state you should be in so that you can get some quality shut eye.

   You don't need to go to bed hungry but avoid eating anything at least 1 hour before bed. This means avoiding late night dinners and especially late night snacks. Your body needs some time to get through the initial stages of digestion before you try to fall asleep.

3. **Stop having cold feet**: no, this doesn't mean you need to resolve any commitment issues you might have, it just means you need to put on a pair of socks.

As your body starts to relax, your circulation slows down and the first parts to suffer are your feet because they are furthest from your heart. In order for your body to get relaxed, it needs to feel warm and cozy. So, slip on a pair of socks if it's particularly cold.

4. **Stop stressing**: this one is definitely easier said than done. But it is worth making the effort. If you're worried about something that is going to happen tomorrow or in the future (or your worried about the consequences of something that did happen), try to think through and find a solution during the day.

When you are trying to fall asleep, stress and worrying are just going to keep you tossing and turning. So, do your best to focus on positive thoughts before bed, knowing that if you wake up feeling refreshed and energized, you have a far better chance of finding a solution than if you are groggy and unable to be fully alert.

If all your best efforts fail and you still find yourself worrying about a problem at night, at least try to focus on thinking about possible solutions rather than just focusing on the negatives and the worst-case scenario.

5. **Stop working in bed**: you need to make sure that your bed is for sleep (and maybe also for making new family members!).

   Don't bring your laptop into bed to study, work, or chat with friends. Your bed is not chair or table. Your bedroom is not a living room.

   You want your body to get the clear message that when you are in bed that means it is time to sleep. If you do anything else in bed, this message won't be clear.

In addition to stopping these bad bedtime habits, you should set up some healthy bedtime habits that will help you fall asleep more easily and get better quality sleep:

1. **Establish a bedtime routine**: you need to have a stable routine that you go through every night before bed. Do the same things in the same order every night. This repetition helps your body realize what's going on.

   If you always brush your teeth, wash your face, and put on pajamas (in that order) before laying down in bed, your body will already know as soon as the toothbrush hits your teeth that it's time to sleep.

   This will help you fall asleep more quickly when you finally lay down. Having this routine also means not doing these things any other time of day (except for brushing your teeth, please brush your teeth more than once a day!).

For example, don't wear pajamas during the daytime. You can have other comfy clothes for a day of relaxing at home but don't wear the same things you wear to bed.

2. **Keep the room cold**: studies have shown that a cold room helps you sleep better than a warm room. This doesn't mean it needs to be freezing but does need to be cooler than usual.

   Your body naturally lowers its temperature while you are sleeping. When the temperature of your room is closer to the temperature that your body is trying to lower to, it will help you get to sleep faster.

   Normally, it is advised to keep the thermostat somewhere between 65 and 72 degrees Fahrenheit. But some people feel more comfortable in lower temperatures (or higher temperatures).

   A good rule of thumb is to lower the temperature about 5 degrees from wherever you like to set it during the day.

3. **Go to bed and wake up at the same time**: this is important for the same reasons that having a steady bedtime routine is important.

   By going to bed at the same time every single night, you are allowing your body to establish a stable biorhythm. It can regulate your hormone cycles so that you get a surge of the hormones that help you wake up in the morning and a surge of the hormones that help you sleep when you are trying to go to sleep.

When you go to bed and wake up at the same time every day, your body learns when to release which hormones. So, avoid pulling any all-nighters and try to wake up at the same time each morning (even if it's a weekend and you could sleep in).

You can't "make up" for lost sleep on the weekends, anyway. That's not how your body works. So, it's more important to keep a stable sleep schedule than to keep changing your bedtime and your wake-up time.

4. **Read a book**: Make sure it's made of paper or it's on an eReader that uses the ink technology to look like real paper instead of having backlight coming out of the screen.

   As mentioned above, you want to avoid screens before bed. If you have trouble keeping your racing thoughts at bay, a book can help distract your mind and make you feel relaxed.

   Get a small book light that you can attach to the book so you can turn off all the other lights and keep the room dark. The darkness will help your body get sleepy and the act of reading will help relax your mind and get it ready for sleep.

If you are liking these tips so far, *you must* check out my 97 weight loss tips that are available to you right here!

If the link is still active, get it while you can, because I will be removing it soon (I can't keep giving away AWESOME secrets like these for free *forever*).

Evening Habit #6 – Cut the Caffeine

A cup of coffee in the morning is a great way to jumpstart your day. The caffeine wakes you up and speeds up your metabolism.

If you drink it without milk or sugar, it is also the ideal zero calorie treat. But beyond 1 or 2 cups in the morning, you should be careful about how much caffeine you consume in a day.

Too much caffeine raises blood pressure, increases anxiety, and can keep you awake at night when you are trying to go to sleep.

Coffee isn't the only source of caffeine. It is also found in soda, tea, chocolate, and even certain pain medications (because it also helps relieve headaches).

So, watch what you eat and drink throughout the day and try to avoid consuming any kind of caffeine at least 4 hours before you plan to go to sleep at night.

Caffeine is a stimulant, which means it keeps your brain awake and alert even when your body is exhausted and ready to call it a day.

Because you need a good, full night of rest every night in order to promote health and weight loss, consuming caffeine to close to your bedtime is going to cause you to gain weight.

In addition to the negative effects of drinking more than 1 or 2 cups of coffee per day, there are a host of other negative health effects to drinking other caffeinated beverages.

The biggest offender is, by far, soda. Regular soda is bad and diet soda is even worse.

Often, soda is loaded with corn syrup or, in the case of diet soda, artificial sweeteners like aspartame.

Your body cannot recognize either of these ingredients and doesn't know how to break them down. So, for lack of any other option, it just stores them as fat.

If you drink soda or consume a lot of foods and beverages that have either corn syrup or an artificial sweetener, this is, undoubtedly, a major factor in any excess weight you have gained.

As soon as you cut these out of your diet, you will notice significant weight loss.

Sodas (whether diet or not) are also very high in sodium. Diets which are high in sodium cause high blood pressure, dehydration, and weight gain.

If you consume too much sodium, your body will start to retain a lot of water which means you'll bloat up with a lot of water weight.

Excess sodium, especially when you are already not drinking enough water every day, also leads to dehydration.

Dehydration causes weight gain, slowed metabolism, as well as many other serious health problems.

So, next time you are feeling thirsty, soda is the absolute last thing you should drink. Rather than quenching your thirst, soda is actually making you *thirstier*.

Too much caffeine can also lead to dehydration because, in addition to being a stimulant, caffeine is also a diuretic.

Diuretics are things that cause you to get rid of more fluid than they add. In the simplest terms, they make you urinate a lot.

You end up expelling more fluids from urination than you took in from drinking the caffeinated beverage. If you don't drink enough water to replace those lost fluids, you will become dehydrated which is extremely unhealthy and also causes weight gain.

So, cut your total caffeine intake to about 200 milligrams per day (or 2 coffee mugs worth of coffee). Cut soda out of your diet entirely.

Action Plan

If you drink coffee in the morning, start decreasing the amount of milk or sugar that you add—if you add any.

Drinking black coffee will give you a stronger effect from the beginning and help you drink less in total. You simply cannot chug a whole cup of hot black coffee.

Without milk to cool it down and sugar to dampen the flavor, you'll be forced to sip slowly and enjoy it at a relaxed pace.

Start cutting out any other caffeine you normally drink after your morning coffee and completely cut out caffeinated beverages 4 hours before you plan to go to sleep.

In the evenings, drink herbal teas that are naturally caffeine free to replace your normal coffee, soda, or black tea. Mint tea is an especially good option because it is naturally caffeine free and the mint will even help you fight cravings.

Remember to drink more water throughout the day as well in order to make sure you are fully hydrated. If you make an effort to stay hydrated throughout the day, you will reduce feelings of fatigue and maintain full alertness.

This means you won't feel the need to get those regular doses of caffeine to keep you going through the day. You need at least 2 liters of water every day.

You can start your day off better by drinking a glass of water with your coffee in the morning. Water in the morning will help wake up your metabolism.

Since coffee is already a metabolism booster, drinking a glass of water with your coffee will act as a double strength boost so you can be sure there is nothing sluggish about your metabolism even if you might still be feeling a little tired in the morning.

As for soda, you should cut this out entirely. If you are a regular soda drinking, this will be more challenging. Soda can be a genuine addiction but it is absolutely worth the struggle.

Even after 1 week of being soda free, you will already notice amazing changes. You'll lose weight, you'll feel more clear-headed and focused, you'll feel more energetic throughout the day rather than experiencing those peaks and crashes of energy that normally come with soda. The list of benefits you'll get from not drinking soda could fill up a book of their own.

If your soda habit is really serious and you actually experience withdrawal-like symptoms, here are a few tips to help you kick the habit:

- **Drink a soda substitute**: buy plain carbonated water and mix it with juice (no sugar added). Alternatively, you can mix it with fresh fruits.

  Berries are an especially delicious option. It won't be a perfect imitation of soda because it is caffeine free, sodium free, and without any added sugar.

  However, it has that carbonated feel that you look for in a can of soda and it will have some sweetness from the juice or fruit that you add.

  So, it allows you to sort of go through the motions of drinking soda and get the experience without getting the added weight and other health problems.

- **Go cold turkey**: with some things, you can cut them out gradually. Soda is not one of those things. It is better to go cold turkey.

  This might sound painful at first but it will make the process of breaking the habits go much more quickly. So, decide today to stop drinking soda and give it up entirely. Don't make excuses.

- **Throw out all the soda in your house**: if there is soda in your house, you are going to drink it. That's all there is to it.

  It's like a smoker who keeps a pack of cigarettes in her purse and says, "I'm not going to smoke them. I'm just hanging on to them."

  If your children or partner also drink soda, tell them they are quitting the habit too. It is better for their health. Plus, making sure that nobody else has soda in the house will help you stay away from the stuff yourself. Your kids might get mad at you but let them get mad.

  They will thank you later when they grow up without diabetes, obesity, or any other health problem that soda causes.

- **Take it one day at a time**: don't try to focus on how hard it is going to be to never drink soda again.

First of all, it is not going to be that hard. After the first 30 days, you'll already find it easier to go without it.

Give it another 30 days after that and you'll already find yourself going a whole week without ever even thinking about it.

Secondly, worrying about the road ahead will only make it more difficult to navigate the road right in front of you. Track your progress and take pride in every single day that you go without soda. Just focus on getting through the next 24 hours. When you've gotten through that, focus on getting through the next 24 hours.

- **Don't beat yourself up**: when you first try to kick the soda habit, you are going to slip up. You're going to have cravings you simply cannot resist.

Fight these cravings with everything you've got. But when you cave in and have a soda, don't feel like it was all a waste of your effort. And don't feel like you are too weak to get through this.

You have still come a long way and you are still further than you were when you started. Most importantly, you can still get right back up and keep going.

Think of it this way: if you normally drink about 2 sodas every day and after doing a 30-day soda free challenge, you slipped up 5 times, that would still be 50 sodas that you *didn't* drink!

That is fantastic progress. The next 30 days will be that much easier because of that accomplishment. Change is not a switch that you flip.

It is a journey that you have to take. If you feel weak now, remember that nobody is strong enough to make it to the end right when they start.

You gather the strength along the way, with each step that you take, each mistake that you make, and each obstacle that you overcome.

So, kick your soda habit, keep your coffee for the morning, and replace evening caffeine with herbal teas or carbonated water with fruits. This sounds like a lot for one habit but the results are well worth the effort.

If you are liking these tips so far, *you must* check out my 97 weight loss tips that are available to you right here!

If the link is still active, get it while you can, because I will be removing it soon (I can't keep giving away AWESOME secrets like these for free *forever*).

Evening Habit #7 – Avoid Alcohol & Tobacco

Alcohol and tobacco should be kept to a minimum no matter whom you are or what you are trying to accomplish.

In excess, these two can cause extremely serious health problems from liver failure to lung cancer.

So, try to save them for special occasions only and even then, only in moderation.

Beyond the many health problems that are associated with alcohol and tobacco (you probably have already heard and read plenty about each of them), they can also contribute to weight gain.

Let's start with tobacco. The nicotine in tobacco acts as a stimulant. That is, it keeps you awake and alert.

In excess, this can cause heightened anxiety and stress (which smokers usually try to fight by smoking more, resulting in even worse anxiety and stress).

If you smoke within 1 to 2 hours of going to bed, you will have a more difficult time falling asleep because your brain is still simulated and alert from the nicotine.

As you already know by now, a lack of quality sleep can have serious consequences on your health and your weight. So, if you are a smoker and don't have any intention of quitting, you should, at the very least, avoid smoking 1 hour before you plan to go to sleep.

You should actually also consider quitting entirely but that is a topic for another book. Try to cut your overall total down to 10 cigarettes per day in order to minimize the anxiety and stress that smoking causes.

Now let's take a look at the weight gain effects of alcohol.

First of all, alcoholic drinks are deceptively high in calories, especially if you are partial to those fancy, sugary cocktails. If you've ever heard someone mentioning "beer bellies", you should know that they are a very real thing.

To give you an idea: one margarita has 153 calories, 12 ounces of beer averages about 150 to 200 calories, and a single shot of tequila will pack 96 calories. That means a night of drinking could end up adding more calories than you ate the entire day!

Opting for the low calorie or light options isn't going to help you much, either.

Like caffeine, alcohol is also a diuretic, causing you to expel more water than you take in from drinking it. It is a more powerful diuretic than caffeine, too.

This is one of the main reasons you get a hangover after a night of drinking. An 8 oz alcoholic beverage will cause you to expel about 33 oz of water!

So, if you aren't drinking water by the gallon as you drink alcohol, you are on the road to severe dehydration.

As you already know, chronic dehydration is one of the factors that contribute to weight gain.

One night of drinking can set you back pretty far. So far, alcohol packs on a ridiculous amount of calories and causes severe dehydration.

But alcohol leads to weight gain in another, less well known way as well. When you consume alcohol, your body switches gears. It is not possible for your body to store any excess alcohol as fat so it has to burn up all the calories as they come in.

This means that the fat burning process that your body typically goes through during the entire day comes to a complete stop.

It even stops metabolizing the other things in your stomach because it is entirely focused on dealing with the alcohol.

So, alcohol is a fat building offender on 3 fronts: it adds calories, it dehydrates you, and it completely stops your body from burning fat.

Action Plan

If you are planning to go out drinking, drink a tall glass of water between each alcoholic beverage you have.

This will not only help replace some of the lost water but will also slow down your drinking and help you drink less.

When you get home, chug a liter of water before bed. You can also try to get a jump-start by drinking more than your usual 2 liters during the day.

Try to drink double the amount of water before you start, continue to drink water as you drink alcohol, and end the night with a lot of water.

This will help prevent dehydration but it won't get rid of the calories. For those, you'll have to get in some serious dancing during the night!

If you aren't going out to drink but you would like to have some wine or beer at home, drink it with dinner and keep it down to 1 or 2 glasses.

Your body needs 1 hour to fully metabolize 1 portion of alcohol. For reference, 1 portion is equal to a 5 oz glass of wine, a 12 oz bottle of beer, or a 1.5 oz shot of hard liquor.

This means you shouldn't drink too close to bed time because you want to give your body the full amount of time it needs to metabolize the alcohol before you go to sleep.

While you may think that alcohol helps you sleep, this is only partially true. It does help you fall asleep more quickly but it prevents your body from going to REM sleep (the most restful kind of sleep). So your overall quality of sleep is poorer if you have alcohol in your system.

With that in mind, it is okay to have that glass or two of wine with your dinner but make sure you have dinner early enough that you have enough hours left before bed to fully metabolize the alcohol.

During those hours that you are metabolizing, drink enough water to replace the total amount of fluid lost from alcohol. For every ounce of alcohol you drank, you need to drink 4 ounces of water.

As for smoking: don't have a cigarette within one hour before you plan to go to bed and try to keep your daily total down to 10 cigarettes.

This will help reduce the impact smoking has on your sleep quality and lower your overall stress levels throughout the day.

A Special Gift Just For YOU

FOR A LIMITED TIME ONLY – Get Linda's best-selling book *"Quick & Easy Weight Loss: 97 Scientifically Proven Tips Even For Those With Busy Schedules!"* absolutely FREE!

Readers who have read this bonus book along with this book have seen the greatest changes in their weight loss both *FAST & EASILY* and have improved overall fitness levels – so it is *highly recommended* to get this bonus book.

Once again, as a big thank-you for downloading this book, I'd like to offer it to you *100% FREE for a LIMITED TIME ONLY!*

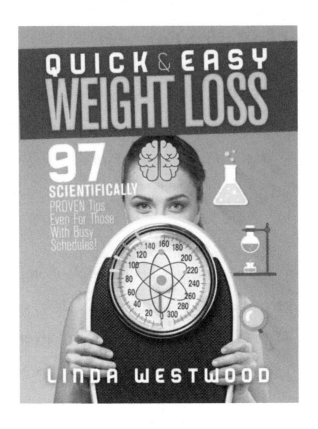

Get your free copy at:

TopFitnessAdvice.com/Bonus

Evening Habit #8 – This Will STOP Evening Food Cravings

If you've already eaten dinner and you still have the urge to munch on something, it is mostly likely because your dinner wasn't satisfying enough.

Later on, in this book, you'll learn more about how to make a satisfying dinner that will help stop cravings before they even start.

But, if a satisfying, balanced dinner still can't kill the cravings, try brushing your teeth.

This probably sounds a little odd. But it actually works.

After brushing your teeth, you won't want to eat anything because the minty flavor won't mix well with food.

Toothpaste and barbecue flavored chips?

No, thank you.

Plus, who wants to ruin freshly cleaned teeth with junk food?

You actually need to wait 30 minutes after brushing your teeth to eat anyway because you need to give the enamel coating on your teeth time to harden again.

Brushing your teeth is also effective because the mint in the toothpaste acts as a craving-fighter. Mint is often used to help stave off strong cravings and control appetite.

Action Plan

Try brushing your teeth right after dinner so that you will be less likely to snack throughout the night.

Alternatively, you can wait about an hour after dinner or whenever the cravings really start to kick in.

To be most effective, you should do it before the cravings truly start. Try to estimate about how long after dinner you get the urge to start snacking and brush your teeth about 5 to 10 minutes before that time.

Evening Habit #9 – Don't Confuse Thirst for Hunger

Recent studies show that as much as 75% of Americans may be suffering from chronic dehydration. That figure is staggering. That means that 3 out of every 4 people in the United States are chronically dehydrated!

Now, your first thought might be, "okay, that is definitely shocking but what exactly does that have to do with losing weight?"

The answer is: everything.

Chronic dehydration causes our bodies to lose the ability to recognize when we are thirsty (which leads to further dehydration). In fact, our thirst receptors are so low that we often confuse thirst for hunger.

For example, if you've ever started to feel a little weak or gotten a headache and thought, "oh, I should probably eat something", you are probably wrong.

Most of the time, these symptoms are signs that your body needs water—no, not soda, not sugary juice, not coffee. It needs water.

Without water, your body simply cannot function. Your body is 60% water. You need it to lubricate your brain, your muscles, your digestive system, and literally everything else.

If you are not drinking at least 2 liters of water per day, you are not drinking enough water.

Chronic dehydration can actually lead to weight gain in addition to a dizzying list of other problems. It leads to digestive disorders, bladder problems, kidney problems, constipation, fatigue and a lot of other health issues that end up causing you to store more fat in the body instead of efficiently burning it off as energy.

Being dehydrated can also lead to irresistible cravings for sugary foods. This is because dehydration means your body doesn't have the water it needs to release glycogen, which is needed to stabilize the glucose levels in your blood.

Blood glucose is what your body uses as energy. When your glucose levels are low, you start craving sweets because sugar can be turned into glucose quickly. If you're dehydrated, you don't actually need to rely on sugar, you just need to drink water so that you can use the energy stores you already have in you.

Water has so many amazing benefits for weight loss, health, and appearance that it's amazing we aren't all guzzling it down on a regular basis.

Here are a few of the benefits of staying thoroughly hydrated:

- **Decrease calories**: water is a zero-calorie method to fighting cravings. As mentioned earlier, most people confuse the signs of dehydration with the signs of hunger and end up eating when a glass of water would actually be more satisfying for your body.

- **Boost metabolism**: water in your body is like oil in your car's engine. It keeps things running smoothly and that includes your digestive system. Your stomach is able to breakdown nutrients more easily and your body can transport those nutrients to the rest of your body more quickly.

- **Clears skin**: drinking enough water helps prevent your pores from getting clogged and reduces the appearance of wrinkles by increasing skin elasticity. This means you'll have smoother, less pimply skin without having to follow some elaborate skin care routine.

- **Improve focus and alertness**: dehydration slows the brain down along with the rest of the body. Some studies have shown that a glass of water could actually be more effective than a cup of coffee when it comes to making you feel more alert, awake, and ready to concentrate on the task at hand.

- **Prevents constipation**: as mentioned earlier, staying hydrated helps to keep things running smoothly. In fact, one of the leading causes of constipation is dehydration. So to avoid getting backed up, make sure you are drinking enough water every day.

Action Plan

The best way to make sure you are hydrated is pretty simple: drink water.

And when I say drink water, I really mean water, not juice or coffee and *especially* not soda.

Cut down on the amount of beverages you buy so that when you are at home, your only real option for drinking is water.

You might think water is plain and boring but it is a completely nonnegotiable necessity. You need to drink 2 liters of water every single day.

Get a water bottle (preferably metal or glass) and figure out how many times you need to refill to make your 2-liter requirement.

For example, if you've got a 1-liter bottle, you'll only need to drink 2 full bottles. Keep this water bottle with you and drink regularly throughout the day.

When you are feeling a little sleepy, drink water. When you are starting to feel a craving for snacks come on, drink water.

In addition to drinking water all throughout the day, you should drink water with every meal. Don't eat without having some water to wash it down.

You can even use water to help slow your pace which, as you have already learned, is another healthy weight loss habit you should practice. Take a sip of water after swallowing each bite to help you eat fewer total calories and help your digestive system break down the food more easily.

Evening Habit #10 – The CURE to Night Binges Fits in Your Pocket!

One of the reasons we enjoy snacking at night so much is because it keeps our body busy while we are watching TV. Even if you aren't actually hungry, you just enjoy chewing while you watch your favorite show.

To get the satisfaction of chewing and help fight cravings, you can try chewing sugarless mint gum.

The mint (as you learned earlier in this book) will help fight your cravings while the act of chewing will keep you busy as you watch TV or surf the internet.

Action Plan

When you get the urge to snack after dinner, try chewing a piece of sugarless mint gum instead.

Buy a bulk package of it and keep it at home so that you'll always have gum as an option to avoid snacking.

It's a good way to trick yourself and avoid packing on calories.

Evening Habit #11 – Take an After Dinner Walk

As you'll learn in the next chapter, watching TV is a major contributor to weight gain. Countless studies have been done on the links between TV and obesity and what they have found is surprising (you'll get the specific numbers in the next chapter).

Not only is it a sedentary activity that doesn't help you burn off calories, it is a major trigger for snacking. If you have trouble avoiding those snacks after dinner, try going for a walk.

Walks burn calories, reduce cravings, decrease stress, and get you out of the house so you don't spend as much time sitting around.

It can also boost your metabolism in a few different ways. For one, exercise triggers your metabolism and revs it up into a higher gear. But walking also decreases stress.

You might remember from the first chapter (about eating slowly and enjoying your food) about how stress causes your metabolism to slow down. It redirects the calories to be stored as fat.

So, a nice walk after dinner can really get your metabolism going to help you burn off extra calories. A brisk 30-minute walk will burn around 150 calories.

At the same time, you'll be out of the house and away from the temptation to start munching. So, add the calories you burned to the number of calories you *didn't* eat and you'll really start to see some change.

There are also a lot of other benefits to walking that go beyond weight loss:

- **Heart health**: daily walks can reduce your bad cholesterol and increase your good cholesterol. It also helps keep blood pressure under control. That same brisk 30-minute walk that's burning 150 calories for you will also reduce your risk for heart disease and stroke by 27%!

- **Prevent disease**: walking can also decrease your risk for type 2 diabetes, certain cancers, and even asthma attacks. In fact, one study showed that people who made a daily habit of walking had a 20% lower risk of getting breast cancer, colon cancer, and cancer of the uterus. So, every woman should make a point to walk at least 30 minutes per day.

- **Increase muscle mass**: walking is a form of exercise so it helps you build muscle. You won't become an international bodybuilding champion but you'll see some welcome muscle tone in your legs and stomach. Plus, the more muscle you have, the more calories you burn (because muscles need more calories to operate than fat).

So, this is yet another weight loss benefit you can get from taking an after-dinner walk.

- **Avoid dementia**: as you age, there are a whole range of new diseases you'll have to start worrying about. About 1 in every 14 people over the age of 65 already has dementia. That jumps to 1 in every 6 people for people over 80. However, walking keeps your brain healthy and strong. Long term studies have shown that people who take walks every day were 40% less likely to show signs of dementia when they got older. This is because walking prevents brain shrinkage which tends to happen as you age.

- **Maintain strong bones**: in addition to dementia, you'll also have to start thinking about osteoporosis when you hit your golden years. As you age, your bone density begins to decrease. This is especially the case if you snack on a lot of calcium-poor junk food and don't get any exercise. So, in addition to getting more calcium in your diet, you should start walking daily to keep your bones strong and prevent osteoporosis in old age.

- **Boost your energy**: if you're feeling lazy or lack motivation, then forcing yourself to go for a walk can give you that surge of energy you need to power through a late-night project or even just feel better in general. It improves your circulation, increases your oxygen supply and keeps you feeling alert. It'll help stretch out stiff joints and reduce muscle pain. So, if you've been sitting all day, a walk is the perfect thing to get rid of that aching, sluggish feeling you get from sitting around for too long.

- **Improve your mood**: moderate exercise of all kinds (and this includes walking) releases neurotransmitters in your brain that allow you to feel pleasure. This can decrease depression, anxiety, and stress. As you already learned, stress slows the metabolism down and pleasure speeds it up. So not only will you feel better, you'll be helping your metabolism out as well! Who knew just being happy could help you lose weight?

After reading about all these benefits, you're probably ready to start making walking part of your evening routine.

Here are a few tips to help you stick with it.

Action Plan

Don't accept excuses.

As soon as you clear the table after dinner, put on your walking shoes and get outside. You might be feeling lazy while you're inside the house but as soon as you get out of the front door and you take your first breath of cool, evening air, you'll be ready to go.

So just skip all the excuses and put on those shoes already!

If you've got a family, have them join you. An evening walk is a great family activity no matter what age your kids are. Even if you've got an infant, pushing the stroller will just lead to more calories burned!

Plus, if your little one has a tough time falling asleep, a ride in the stroller will usually help them pass right out. You'll be helping yourself lose weight and instilling the right habits in your children for when they get older.

If you've got a pet, going for a walk will be even more fun (assuming your pet is not a goldfish, that is). Your dog's motivation and excitement about going for a walk will help you get motivated yourself.

After a few days of nightly walks, your dog will push you to stick with the habit even on the evenings when you're having doubts. And how can you say no to that adorable puppy face?

If you don't have pet, consider getting one! Not only will they get you up and walking, they decrease stress, which, as you know, is a great boost to your weight loss efforts.

Whether you are walking alone or walking with family, the trick is to just do it. Don't do any other activity after dinner before you have taken your walk. It should just become an automatic part of dinner time. You haven't finished until you've gotten back from your walk.

As soon as you turn on the TV or start surfing the internet, it's going to be a lot harder to motivate yourself to get out the door. So, walk first, be lazy later.

The bottom line is you just need to start walking!

30 minutes after dinner of walking is all it takes to get the full range of benefits that walking has to offer.

That's 30 minutes of getting exercise, boosting your metabolism, decreasing stress, decreasing disease, burning calories, and countless other things. No TV show, no matter how good, can offer you those kinds of benefits!

Evening Habit #12 – Turn off the T.V.

If you have ever in your life eaten food purely out of boredom, then you already know the dangers of letting your mind or body get bored.

While the television might seem like a cure for boredom, it's more of a distraction from the bored feeling. It doesn't stimulate your mind or get your body moving. It just flashes some nice colors and sounds at you so you don't have to think about boredom.

To kill boredom, you need activities that actually require some thinking or physical action—or both!

One of the reasons snacking goes so well with watching TV is that your body is just desperate for something to do instead of just sitting there.

You need to add more stimulating activities to your evening schedule to keep your mind off that package of string cheese in the fridge that's calling your name.

The average American watches 5 hours of television every day. This fact alone is enough to decide that you should cut down on the amount of television.

You could use that time to do so many other enjoyable things. But if you combine that with the fact the average personal also eats between 100 and 300 calories during 1 hour of watching television, the numbers become even more shocking.

Think of how much weight you could lose just by cutting out one hour of TV per day?

That would be 7 hours less per week, which could work out to as much as 2,100 fewer calories per week depending on how much you snack while in front of the TV.

If you cut TV out entirely, and replace it with something healthy, such as walking, you could flip your calories in/out balance for the entire week by up to 5,000 calories!

The numbers are staggering. So, it's worth dropping your television time and finding a better way to relax when you get home from work in the evening.

Action Plan

Try reading a book. It's got characters, plots, and drama just like your TV shows but it requires more brain activity because you have to actively read the words on the page and then interpret the meaning of the words and the sentence as a whole.

Of course, you don't consciously think about interpreting the meaning but your brain is doing it.

The reason it doesn't do the same thing when you've got the TV on is because the images on the screen already do half the work for you.

You don't have to imagine what the characters look like, how they said something, what their voice might look like, or even what the background setting looks like when it's all already there on the screen.

When your brain is busy using imagination, it's going to spend less time imagining the snacks in your kitchen.

If you're not a huge fan of reading (with the exception of this book, at least), my first suggestion is to give it another chance. There are so many books out there that you are bound to find something that sparks your interest.

And in this age of eBooks, you have easy access to millions of books.

But if you are still reluctant to choose a book over the TV, try other activities.

Get crafty by making your own jewelry, soaps, clothes, or literally anything else. Learn a new language or practice a new skill. Have a game night with the family or take up gardening. Start painting or drawing.

In fact, here are dozens of things that you can do instead of snacking to take your mind off the munchies:

- Light some scented candles and take a long, hot bath
- Invite your partner into the tub with you!
- Organize your home office or your closet
- Try knitting or crocheting
- Treat yourself to a spa evening: facials, manicures, the whole nine yards

- Put on your favorite music and dance
- Have an impromptu dance party with the whole family!
- Invite your friends while you're at it!
- Start keeping a journal and write in it
- Go through old pictures and reminisce
- Annoy your pets
- Water your plants (alternatively: buy some plants. Then water them)
- Get rid of clothes you don't want
- Go shopping to replace the clothes you got rid of
- Learn to play an instrument
- Call a friend or relative to chat
- Play solitaire (like, with actual cards)
- Build a house out of cards (then knock it over when you get frustrated with them)
- Plan a weekend trip for the family (or a weekend getaway with your friends)
- Find creative new uses for things in your house
- Make sock monkeys with the kids
- Actually try one of those cool ideas you saw on the internet
- Do something that you have been procrastinating on for too long

There are hundreds of things you can do instead of watch TV. This doesn't mean you have to throw out your television. Just only watch it when you have a specific show you enjoy watching.

Then, turn it off when it's over and do something else. If you ever catch yourself flipping through the channels to see what's on, that's the sign it's time to turn it off and do something else.

Once you get into the habit of doing other things aside from watching TV, not only will you keep yourself distracted from snacking, you'll also free up a lot of time to do activities that are way more rewarding.

You're going to wonder why you ever wasted so much time flipping through channels to look for something that was at least moderately entertaining.

There's a whole wide world out there (or even a whole wide house out there) that's waiting for you to explore its opportunities. You'll be able to have more quality time with your loved ones and build lasting memories.

When you do decide to turn on the TV, do something else instead of snacking.

For example, watching TV can be the perfect time to power through some crunches or if your living room is big enough, put a treadmill in there and go for a run while watching your favorite show.

If you are liking these tips so far, *you must* check out my 97 weight loss tips that are available to you right here!

If the link is still active, get it while you can, because I will be removing it soon (I can't keep giving away AWESOME secrets like these for free *forever*).

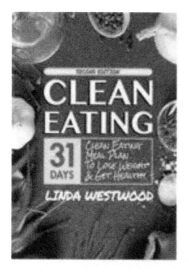
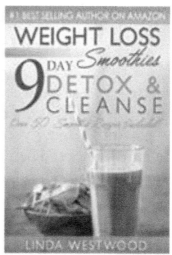
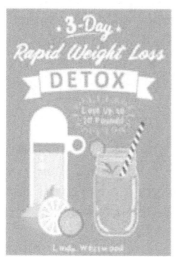
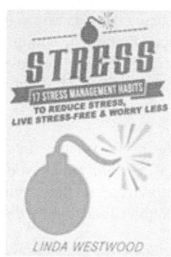

Check out Linda's best selling books at:

TopFitnessAdvice.com/go/books

Evening Habit #13 – Curb Cravings with Nutrition (Part I)

The battle against between meal cravings begins with nutrition. If you get all the nutrients you need from your 3 main meals of the day, your body simply won't have any need to crave snacks in between.

Your cravings are not some mysterious part of your subconscious mind; it's a simple matter of your body feeling like it doesn't have enough.

Of course, there is some psychology to it. Some people practice "emotional eating." That is, they eat in order to avoid dealing with negative emotions. This is where the cliché of eating a big tub of ice cream after a breakup comes from.

But the primary factor in cravings is poor nutrition so if you eat a healthy diet, you won't have as many between meal cravings and the cravings you do have will start to be for healthier foods rather than junk and sweets.

So, in part I, we are going to focus on fiber.

Fiber is a powerful tool against weight loss. It helps you feel fuller and it is a huge boost to your metabolism. In fact, if you ate absolutely no fiber, you wouldn't be able to digest food.

Your body needs fiber in order to push the food through your whole system and finally expel it.

Because fiber takes more time to break down than sugars and other junk foods, it keeps you feeling full and satisfied for a lot longer and adds a lot less calories.

It also stabilizes your glucose levels because it acts as a shield that slows your body's absorption of glucose. So, it stabilizes the rate at which your body gets the energy from your food instead of just sending it all as one big burst at the beginning.

This means you avoid the peak and crash cycle that comes with a high sugar diet.

Fiber also helps control your appetite because, although it is low in calories, it is a really bulky form of nutrition.

It takes up a lot of space in the stomach and moves slowly throughout your digestive system so you end up feeling full after eating less.

Fiber is what gives vegetables their crispy texture and whole grain breads their full-bodied flavor. Fiber is why a spoonful of peanut butter feels a lot more satisfying and filling than a spoonful of jelly.

It is also what helps you digest and use the other nutrients in your food.

Studies have shown that fiber improves your body's ability to absorb minerals like calcium, zinc, and magnesium. So, if you take a daily supplement, make sure you eat a high fiber meal with it so you can make sure your body absorbs as much as possible.

Action Plan

Include more fiber in your diet throughout the day but also at dinnertime.

At dinner, you want to try and get your fiber from low carbohydrate foods. As you read earlier in this book, cutting down on carbohydrates at dinnertime is a great strategy for losing weight.

If you're coming up short on answers for foods that are high in fiber but also low in carbohydrates, here are some ideas for you:

- **Avocado**: an avocado is a nutrition goldmine. It's full of vitamins and minerals your body needs and it also happens to be delicious. Plus, it's got healthy, unsaturated fat which you want to add in your dinner. Plus, one avocado has just 3 grams of carbohydrates but offers 12 grams of fiber. So, it is a great option for a low carbohydrate dinner.

- **Broccoli**: this is another great low carbohydrate option for dinner. One cup of chopped, cooked broccoli yields 16 grams of fiber with only 6 grams of carbohydrates. So, load up on broccoli for a nutritious, filling, low carbohydrate meal.

- **Cauliflower**: broccoli's tasty cousin is also a great low carbohydrate dinner option. One cup of these provides 4 grams of fiber with just 2 grams of carbohydrates. So, combine it with broccoli for a colorful, low carbohydrate plate.

- **Collard greens**: in one cup of cooked, chopped collard greens, you'll get 5 grams of fiber but only 4 grams of carbohydrates. You can stir these up into almost anything to add some nice texture and flavor to any meal.

In general, when you are looking for a low carbohydrate, high fiber food, you want to look for vegetables that aren't too starchy.

Potatoes and corn are good examples of extremely starchy foods that you'll want to try and keep off your dinner plate. Although, you can welcome them onto your lunch plate!

Aside from the low carbohydrate options above, beans, legumes, and whole grains are fantastic sources of fiber that also boast a high amount of protein as well.

So, you can kill two birds with one nutritious stone if you add these to your meal.

Actually, since they are also loaded with other vitamins and minerals, it's more like killing dozens of birds with one stone.

Evening Habit #14 – Curb Cravings with Nutrition (Part II)

In part II of our quest to fight cravings with nutrition, we will look at protein.

Protein is a more complex nutrient than you might think. That's because it's not just one nutrient (like fiber or calcium). It's actually 9 separate amino acids that all work together.

The reason you need to know that protein is built up of 9 essential amino acids is because not all protein sources contain the same amino acids.

For example, if you tried to live entirely on beans as your protein source, you would become deficient in 2 of the essential amino acids that you need because beans don't provide you with all nine.

Fish, beef, chicken, and all other animal sources of protein do provide a complete spectrum of all 9 essential amino acids but if you ate exclusively beef as your source of protein, you'd get the high blood pressure and high cholesterol that come with it. So, it is important to eat a range of protein sources.

For most plant sources of protein, you'll need to combine different sources to get all 9 essential amino acids.

For example, if you eat beans, combine it with rice or corn. Rice and corn each have a higher amount of the 2 amino acids that beans are lacking while beans have a high supply of the amino acids that both rice and corn are lacking.

You can also combine nuts and seeds with quinoa to create another delicious (and complete) protein.

Now, let's talk about how protein helps you lose weight. Usually when we think about fat burning diets, meat, beans, and nuts don't usually come to mind.

These are rich, flavorful foods and diets usually demand that we get rid of flavor and suffer through our days surviving on plain lettuce.

Eating only lettuce will make you lose weight but there's no reason to suffer when you can lose just as much weight while eating a delicious and healthy diet.

Protein is essential to that healthy, weight loss diet. This is because protein takes a long time for your body to break down and absorb.

The longer it takes food to move through your digestive system, the longer you will feel full.

Protein is, by far, the most difficult thing for your system to process so it spends the longest amount of time in your stomach. This will keep you feeling completely full all the way to your next meal.

Because it also absorbs into your system more slowly, your blood glucose levels are stabilized so you don't experience a sudden crash.

Sudden drops in the amount of glucose in your blood are a major cause of cravings. By avoiding the crash, you avoid the cravings that come with it.

Action Plan

You want to eat a lot of protein at dinner. By a lot, we are talking about 25 grams. This is the number one way to stave off late night cravings.

Protein combined with low carbohydrate sources of fiber and unsaturated fats will keep your blood glucose levels as stabilized as possible while also keeping you feeling full.

This means that your dinner will attack the two main causes of after dinner snacking.

Good sources of protein include fish, poultry, chicken, beans, legumes, nuts, and seeds. Remember to combine your plant sources so that you get the full range of protein.

At dinner, your protein source (or sources if you're combining) should be the largest portion on your plate. The second largest should be your unsaturated fats. The smallest portion should be your fiber rich carbohydrates.

If you're eating fish, you don't need to add any other fatty foods because fish are naturally rich in unsaturated fats.

If you're eating beans or legumes, you don't need to add any other fiber sources because these are already high enough in fiber.

As you plan your meals for the week, make sure your dinner is the most protein rich meal of your day. Do this by eating a little less protein during breakfast and lunch so that you don't go overboard.

Remember, you need 50 grams of protein, 30 grams of fiber, and 20 grams of unsaturated fats.

This is, of course, assuming you have no major health conditions that give you special dietary requirements.

By making sure that you choose a variety of foods for each of these three things, you can make sure that you are also getting a good amount of the vitamins and minerals that you need.

In a single day, you should have at least 3 different sources of protein, 3 different sources of fiber, and 3 different sources of fat.

Throughout the week, try to have 5 different sources of each one that you cycle through over the course of your week. This kind of variety not only helps you cover all your vitamins and minerals, it also keeps your diet from getting dull and boring.

Variety is the spice of life, after all.

Evening Habit #15 – Establish Food-Free Zones

One good way to restrict when you eat is to restrict *where* you eat.

When you eat in the living room or bedroom, it makes it easy to just grab a snack and mindlessly munch even when you're not hungry.

We all do it and it seems like a harmless activity but it does actually cause some problems because you aren't paying attention to the signals your body is telling you. The more you ignore those "I've had enough" signals from your stomach, the more your body will start to ignore them, too.

This makes it harder and harder to avoid overeating.

By restricting the places in your house where food is allowed, you can make sure that you are always consciously deciding when you eat and how much you eat.

You will become more aware of when you start to feel full and should stop. You'll also be able to actually enjoy the flavors more and avoid letting a whole bar of chocolate disappear without you even realizing you ate it all. Plus, it will mean no more crumbs on the bed or sofa!

Part of the logic behind this habit is that you have fewer opportunities to be distracted while eating. When you eat in the living room, it's usually because you are watching TV or surfing the Internet.

On the other hand, if you had to get up from the couch and go to the kitchen every time you wanted to eat a handful of popcorn, you will be much less likely to snack.

So, choosing one or two places in the house where food is allowed will make sure that you snack less and that you can make smarter choices about what you eat.

You'll be paying more attention to the food and more attention to what your body is telling you, which will also help you recognize when you are full and avoid overeating.

With that in mind, not just snacks but all your meals during the day should be eaten in the same place. Adopting this habit will reprogram your brain and body to know when it's time to eat. Once it becomes a habit, you will retrain your subconscious to associate that one place with eating. This will help regulate and moderate your appetite so that you only start to feel hungry when it's actually time to eat. You'll have fewer between meal cravings.

This is the same logic behind evening habit #5 (make sleep a priority). Part of preparing for sleep is not doing other activities in the bed (like eating, watching TV, or working).

This helps your subconscious realize that when it is in bed, it is time to go to sleep. The same thing is happening when you associate eating with only certain areas in the house.

Action Plan

The most logical place to eat is the kitchen or dining room. Your food-free zones should be absolutely everywhere else in the house.

Don't bring food in the living room, bedroom, bathroom, laundry room, garage, or anywhere else. Prepare your meals in the kitchen and eat them sitting down at the table.

While you are eating, don't watch TV or use the computer. Pay attention to your food. Eat slowly and savor the flavors. Make sure that you are sitting down while you eat.

When you stand and eat, your body is in a constant state of feeling like it should be on the go.

This makes it more difficult to eat slowly and focus only on eating. So, sit down, take your time, and let meal time be a relaxing activity. Don't let it be a rushed or stressful part of your day.

When you're done, clear the dishes and continue with your night.

Doing anything else while you eat will lower your ability to recognize when you feel full.

This means you'll have a tendency to overeat because you're just shoveling in food without giving your body the time it needs to send the signal to your brain that it's full.

The second part of this habit is not using the kitchen or dining room for any other activity. If you have limited space in your home and you can't avoid using the dining table for other purposes as well, that's okay.

Just make sure you don't do those other activities at the same time you are eating. If you can avoid it, though, it's best to make your kitchen and dining room "food-only" zones while the rest of your house becomes a "food-free" zone.

At work, avoid eating at your desk if you can. Use the break room or eat your lunch outside.

Don't snack while you work. If you need to eat a snack, leave your desk to do it. Just like at home, your workspace should be a food-free zone.

If your schedule allows for it, make sure you eat your meals in these places at the same time each day or at least within 30 minutes to an hour of a set time.

The more structured your eating habits become, the less likely you will be to have sporadic cravings. Your stomach (well, technically, your subconscious) will learn that if it's not 7pm and you're not in the dining room, then it's not time to be hungry.

This might be tough if you have kids who are used to snacking in front of the TV but remain firm. If you do, not only can you help yourself break this bad habit, you'll be helping your kids to build up these good, healthy habits now while they are still young.

You'll thank yourself next time you're doing the dishes and you don't have to run all around the house looking for stray cups and plates.

Not to mention you'll no longer have to deal with all the spills and stains on carpets, tables, and floors!

Well, except in the kitchen or dining room, that is.

Evening Habit #16 – Know What Your Body Is Actually Telling You

The bad news is a craving for gummy bears doesn't mean your body is dangerously low on Vitamin Gummy.

The good news is you can kill that gummy bear craving by eating a healthy alternative.

You don't have to suffer through sweet tooth withdrawals if you know what your cravings actually mean. Eating a nutritious snack that provides the nutrients your body actually needs will get rid of that unhealthy craving and leave you feeling even more satisfied (and a whole lot less guilty!).

Cravings are not just random impulses to eat a certain food. They are actually signals your body is sending you to let you know what nutrients it's running low on at the moment.

Unfortunately, the signal gets lost in translation very easily especially if you are used to a diet high in junk food. Your body can't tell you exactly what food it needs; all it can do is make you crave a certain range of flavors.

That means it is up to you to decode the message and figure out what your cravings really mean.

Each craving you have is a sign that you are low on a specific nutrient (or set of nutrients).

By snacking on foods that contain those nutrients, you can get rid of the unhealthy craving that is making you suffer, give your body what it really needs, and keep your calories down in a healthy range all at the same time.

Action Plan

Put this knowledge to use by figuring out exactly which healthy foods will help fight which cravings and buying those healthy alternatives at the store instead of buying the unhealthy snacks you usually get.

To help you correctly translate your cravings and find the healthy snack alternatives that will help you get rid of them, here is a quick chart that you can keep for easy reference:

What Your Craving:	What You Actually Need:	What You Should Eat:
Sugary Foods and Sweets	+ Chromium + Phosphorus + Tryptophan + Glucose (i.e.- you may have low blood sugar)	Nuts, seeds, beans, legumes, fresh fruit, eggs, dairy (High protein or natural sugars to stabilize glucose levels and restore nutrients)
Bready or Starchy Foods	+ Nitrogen	Nuts, beans, legumes, oatmeal, quinoa (High protein

		foods and high fiber foods)
Fatty Foods	+ Healthy, unsaturated fats + Calcium	Fish, nuts, seeds, legumes, beans, yogurt, avocado, broccoli, olive oil (Foods high in unsaturated fats or calcium)
Coffee or Caffeine	+ Phosphorus + Iron + Water (i.e.- you may be dehydrated*)	Nuts, legumes, eggs, poultry, beef, water (Drink water and eat high protein foods since they are also often high in phosphorus and iron)
Alcohol	+ Protein + Calcium + Potassium	Meat, nuts, seeds, legumes, beans, dark leafy greens, bananas, yogurt, squash, oatmeal (High protein foods and high mineral foods)
Carbonated Drinks	+ Calcium	Yogurt, legumes, broccoli, spinach, dark leafy greens,

		canned salmon (with bones), molasses (High calcium foods and also drink water)
Salty Foods	+ B vitamins + Vitamin C + Potassium + Decrease Stress**	Bananas, dark leafy greens, fish, liver, poultry, tomatoes, kiwis (Foods high in B vitamins, Vitamin C, or potassium)
Cigarettes	+ Silicon + Tyrosine	Nuts, seeds, legumes (Mineral rich, hearty foods. Also avoid refined flour, sugar, and starches)
Chocolate	+Magnesium +Glucose (low blood sugar again)	Dark chocolate (70% cocoa), fish, spinach, other dark leafy greens (Foods with high magnesium content)

*If you are craving a cup of coffee because you feel tired or groggy, you may actually be dehydrated. Studies show that drinking a glass or two of water when you hit that mid-afternoon lull could perk you up even more than a cup of coffee. Of course, if you're long time coffee drinker, you are probably also addicted to the caffeine but you should try to have a tall glass of water with your coffee.

**Salty food cravings are almost always a sign of excess stress hormones in the body, so you can also try stress reducing techniques like deep breathing, meditation, or calm walks in the park to reduce this craving.

In addition to cravings, there are a few other symptoms of nutrition deficiency that your body is using to try and tell you to get more of a certain vitamin or mineral.

Here are three of the most common ones:

Symptom:	What You Actually Need:	What You Should Eat:
PMS	+ Zinc + Iron + Folate	Red meats (especially liver and other organ meats), seafood, dark leafy greens, carrots, turnips (High protein foods, especially meat and high fiber foods, especially root vegetables)

Loss of Appetite	+ B Vitamins + Manganese + Chloride	Red meat, nuts, seeds, beans, legumes, fish, blueberries, pineapple (High protein or mineral rich foods. If you also have nausea, try beef broths or fresh pineapple juice mixed with sparkling water)
Overeating, Binge Eating	+ Silicon + Tryptophan + Tyrosine	Nuts, seeds, liver, lamb, spinach, orange/green/red fruits and vegetables (High protein and mineral rich foods, high vitamin C. Also avoid refined flour, sugar, and starches)

The alternative snack options in this chart may not sound like they could possibly satisfy your cravings. I mean, who wants to eat fish when they're really craving donuts?

But this chart is based on the science behind those cravings, not the flavors themselves.

If you want donuts and you opt for a healthy sweet option like dried apricots, you're going to be disappointed. Not only are the apricots not as sugary and fluffy as a donut, they don't have the specific nutrient your body is actually craving.

So, while these foods might sound like they're in a whole different ballpark from your craving, eating them will actually stop the craving and make you feel more satisfied afterward.

It will take some time to adapt to this healthy snacking habit, especially if you have formed an emotional or psychological dependency on the foods your craving.

But if you stick with it and fight your cravings with healthy food, you will eventually reprogram your brain and correct the signal so that when your body is low on a certain nutrient, it can tell you to crave the right foods.

Just watch, in a few weeks, you're going to find yourself actually craving broccoli!

Evening Habit #17 – Make After-Dinner Snacking Hard Work

When you feel like having a snack in the evening, it's very rarely because you are actually hungry. Most of that craving is just a simple habit.

You are used to snacking so you keep snacking. This is especially the case when you are watching TV or doing some other activity while you eat.

It can be comforting or relaxing to just go through the motions of snacking.

You might open a bag of cookies as you turn on the TV and before the first commercial break, it's empty and you hardly even remember eating that many cookies.

It can be difficult to fight the urge to munch while you're watching your favorite show. This is one of the reasons that evening habit #12 is so important (watching less TV).

Cutting down on the amount of TV you watch will help cut down on the amount of TV time snacking you do.

Of course, we all have our shows and no matter how much we want to lose weight, it's not worth giving up our favorite show!

So if you must find out what happens to your favorite characters and you can't resist the urge to snack while you watch, then pick snacks that are hard work.

Slowing down the time between bites gives your body time to react and feel full (as you read in the first chapter). It also lets you indulge in the act of snacking without consuming as many calories since you're not shoveling in bite after bite.

Instead, you're eating at a slow, even pace with plenty of breaks in between.

Action Plan

Instead of cookies, go for pistachios in the shell. The time it takes you to break the shell open will help slow down your eating and cut down on the total amount of calories you consume while watching TV.

Some other good hard-work snacking options include oranges, pomegranates, cherries with the pit in, sunflower seeds in the shell, oranges with the peel on.

You can also get a nutcracker and go for walnuts, pecans, and other shelled nuts. Bringing tools into your snack time will take it to a whole new level!

Another way to make snacking hard work is to take a food that is simple to eat and make it more difficult.

Instead of biting into a whole apple, take a knife with you and cut slices out one at a time. Keep a glass of water with you and take a drink from it between every bite.

Whichever method you choose, make sure your snacks are still healthy.

Eating cookies slowly might mean fewer cookies, but they're still cookies. Try to choose hard-work snacks that are healthy and nutritious like the ones already mentioned above.

Evening Habit #18 – "Serving Size" Is Not Just a Suggestion

This habit sounds simple but it can actually be pretty challenging.

You know that serving size mentioned on the package of your favorite snack?

For a box of cookies, the serving size is probably something like 1 or 2 cookies. Well, when you want to eat a sugary, junky snack, eat only a single serving.

Don't take the whole box of cookies with you, just pull out a single serving.

This will help you cut down on junk food and sweets (and slowly start eliminating them or only eating them on special occasions) without having to totally give it all up at once.

Action Plan

If you have had a craving for chips that's lasted hours and you just don't have the willpower to fight it anymore, go ahead and have some chips.

But first check the packaging to see how many chips are in a single serving.

Remove that amount of chips from the bag and put the rest of the bag away.

Eat your chips slowly, savor them.

Last Chance to Get YOUR Bonus!

FOR A LIMITED TIME ONLY – Get Linda's best-selling book *"Quick & Easy Weight Loss: 97 Scientifically Proven Tips Even For Those With Busy Schedules!"* absolutely FREE!

Readers who have read this bonus book along with this book have seen the greatest changes in their weight loss both *FAST & EASILY* and have improved overall fitness levels – so it is *highly recommended* to get this bonus book.

Once again, as a big thank-you for downloading this book, I'd like to offer it to you *100% FREE for a LIMITED TIME ONLY!*

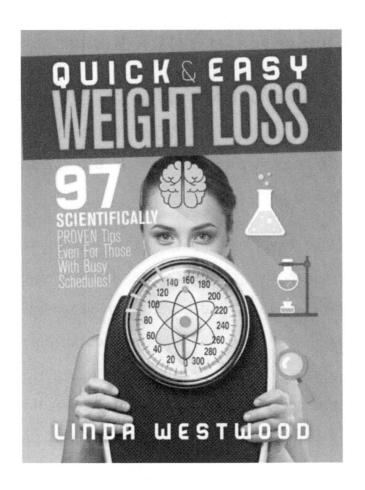

To download your FREE book, go to:

TopFitnessAdvice.com/Bonus

Evening Habit #19 – Start Snack-Free Shopping

The grocery store is where your battle to cut calories begins. Studies have proven that people are more likely to have cravings for foods that are close to them and readily available.

If you know you've got a secret stash of cookies hiding in the kitchen, it's going to take all of your mental energy to resist devouring them.

But if there aren't any cookies to eat, you'll be less likely to have cravings for them.

Of course, you will start to miss them but the craving won't be as strong as if they were in your house, whispering your name, beckoning you to come enjoy just one little bite.

Ban snacks (especially junk food) from your grocery cart and avoid having to face your greatest temptations every night when you get home.

The food that you have in your house should only be ingredients for meals. If it's ready to eat, don't buy it. The exception to that rule is, of course, fruits and vegetables that you can eat raw.

Don't buy chips, cookies, soda, crackers, candy, granola bars, or anything like that. You should even avoid the "healthy" snacks because the goal here is to break your snacking habit.

There are some foods that are ready to eat and totally snack-worthy that you might consider if you've got a serious habit and don't feel like you're ready to give up snacking all at once.

Here is a quick list of foods that burn more calories than they actually contain (because chewing and digesting use up more calories than the amount in the food):

1. **Celery**: if you skip the peanut butter and eat them plain, celery is 75% water and 25% water. Because of this, 1 large stalk (about 12 inches long) contains just 10 calories.

   You'll burn that just from chewing. Even more calories will be burned as you digest it.

   Plus, the high amount of fiber will help you digest and help you feel fuller. It's also full of vitamins. So you can snack totally guilt free.

2. **Grapefruit**: these vitamin-rich gems contain 51 calories, which may sound like you can't burn it all from eating, but grapefruit actually boosts your metabolism!

   Plus, you have to peel it, pull it apart, chew it, and digest it so all the calories burned does add up. The high fiber content will also leave you feeling satisfied while you boost your immune system and lower your cholesterol!

3. **Watermelon**: this fruit is delicious so it probably won't take much convincing to get you to add it to your cart. But you'll be pleased to learn that because watermelon is (not surprisingly) mostly water, it contains very few calories.

   It's also got (more surprisingly) protein. Between the protein and fiber, you'll be able to feel full without adding any calories since digestion burns more than the amount watermelon has to start with.

4. **Broth**: vegetable broth, beef broth, any kind of broth will give you that nice warm, savory flavor you look for in a hearty meal without all the calories that usually come with it.

   So if you must snack after dinner and it must be something substantial, opt for a bowl of warm broth instead.

   The warmth will be soothing, the flavor will satisfy your tongue, and you'll even get some nutrition from it as well!

5. **Apples**: biting, chewing, and digesting an apple all require more calories than you'll actually find in the apple itself.

   They're a sweet, high fiber treat that will fill you up without fattening you up.

Plus, one study showed that eating apples daily could reduce your risk by as much as 17%! It turns out an apple a day really does keep the doctor away.

6. **Chili Peppers**: while you probably don't feel like munching down on a chili pepper by itself, slicing them up and adding them to another snack (or to your main meals) is a great way to boost your metabolism.

    Capsaicin (the compound in peppers that gives them their kick) is scientifically proven to increase metabolism and help you burn more calories.

    Slice them up and mix them into a bowl of vegetables or fruits (sugar and spice are made for each other!). Make a spicy salsa and dollop it on some lettuce for a low calorie, metabolism boosting treat!

7. **Tomatoes**: these are a delicious low calorie option that packs a lot of flavor and a lot of vitamins. Plus, it's the perfect base to that salsa you're going to make!

Action Plan

Make a shopping list before you go to the store. The list should be snack-free, of course!

The best way to make a shopping list is to first plan out all of your meals for the week (or the month, depending on how often you go to the store).

Figure out exactly what ingredients you need and how much of each ingredient you need. Then, when you get to the store, buy only those ingredients and only enough for your meals.

You can actually save a lot of money this way and not just from cutting out snacks. If you plan meals that share ingredients, you can buy some things in bulk and save money.

Plan nutritious meals that are high in fiber and protein so that they keep you feeling full and satisfied even between meals. Don't stress too much about the calorie counts on your main meals.

The most important thing is the nutrition value. If you're getting enough nutrition from your main meals, you'll be less likely to snack in between.

So don't buy low-fat or low-calorie versions of your ingredients. Moderate amounts of unsaturated fats are an important part of a balanced diet and can also help you feel more satisfied after your meal.

Since you'll be cutting out between meal snacks, you can afford to add a few extra calories to your main meals in the name of satisfaction, nutrition and flavor!

To sum it all up, this should be your new grocery shopping routine:

1. Plan all of your meals for the week (breakfast, lunch, and dinner).

a. Make sure they are high fiber, high protein meals made from unprocessed foods

2. Write out a list of all the ingredients

   a. Include the exact amount of each ingredient that you need to make all of your meals

3. Go to the store and buy exactly what is on your list.

   a. No extras and no splurges. Walk right past that snack isle and don't look back!

If you are still not confident that a nutritious meal is enough to get you through the day without snacking, buy some of the options suggested above so that you can snack without adding calories.

Evening Habit #20 – Track Your Progress and Stay Motivated

Tracking your progress is more about making sure you stay on course and don't lose sight of your goals but this is an important part of losing weight.

If you don't keep track of how well you've been doing, you'll be less likely to stick with your weight loss habits in the long run.

Keeping track can also help make sure you don't forget anything. When you are juggling a lot of new habits at once (even if you are doing it one step at a time), it can be difficult to remember all the new things you are doing.

Get a notebook or keep a file on your computer for keeping a daily record of your progress.

You can look through it at the end of each week to see how well you've done, figure out where you might need to make some improvements, and just generally take pride in the fact that you are committing to making this change in your life.

This can be a major source of motivation because in the daily struggle of trying to adopt healthier habits, every little setback might feel like an insurmountable obstacle.

But when you take the time to look back and see that you have actually managed to do surprisingly well (even with a few slip ups here and there), you'll have the encouragement you need to keep going for the next week.

As the weeks add up and you see that you've got over a month of progress recorded, you'll be able to see how far you have actually come.

Habits that seemed completely impossible to keep up with at the beginning could become some of your favorite routines.

Journaling throughout this experience of making healthy changes to your lifestyle is also a great activity to do in the evening.

Not only is it a stimulating activity that will keep you distracted from snacking, it's also a great way to stay motivated even at night (which is when our energy and willpower are usually at their lowest).

Action Plan

Your progress journal can include whatever information you feel is the most important to keep track of but here are some ideas of the sort of things you could include:

- Number of calories you've eaten

- Number of calories burned

- Number of calories you *haven't* eaten

- Amount of weight lost (do this weekly rather than daily)

- Amount of money spent on food

- Amount of money *saved* on food

- Brief descriptions of your mood, energy levels, changes in your physical or emotional wellbeing, or just how you are feeling about the challenge you have chosen to take on

Create a journal entry template with space for each of the things you want to include and fill it out every evening. You can do it as soon as you get home from your post-meal evening walk!

At the end of every week, as you record your new weight, take some time to look back through the records for each day.

You can do a weekly tally of how many calories you didn't eat and write down a few notes about what your goals are for the week ahead.

Create a template for reflecting so that you can make a conscious effort to thoroughly reflect on your progress each week.

Include questions like these:

1. What was my biggest accomplishment last week?

2. What was my greatest challenge last week?

3. Did I meet all of my goals for the week?

4. What do I want to accomplish next week?

5. What might be my greatest challenges next week?

6. What are some strategies I can use to overcome those challenges?

A thorough system for keeping track of your progress will help you stay on track and be a constant source of motivation.

The achievements you have made might not be easy to notice as they happen gradually from day to day but when you have them written down on paper, you will be surprised how far you have come in such a short amount of time.

Evening Habit #21 – Take the 30-Day Weight Loss Challenge

This last habit is not so much a daily habit as a way for you to adopt the other 20 habits you have read about in this book.

By slowly adding in these healthy habits, you can help make sure that you don't lose focus or motivation. Some of these are big changes and when you combine them all, that's a dramatic change to your current lifestyle.

If you attempted to do it all at once, you'd find it impossible to juggle them all and lose hope pretty quickly.

You can create your own 30-day challenge that works better for you but the plan suggested here is an effective way to help you adopt each habit and make sure that it sticks.

Tweak the plan as needed to suit your own situation but don't overburden yourself. Also, don't make it too easy on yourself. This is going to be a challenge no matter how you tackle it. So, find a good, steady pace that works for you.

This 30-day weight loss challenge is not meant to help you lose all the weight in 30 days and then go back to your old lifestyle.

These are habits you should keep for a lifetime so that the weight comes off and stays off for good. If you stick to it, you will notice dramatic results after your first 30 days.

You are going to lose a lot of water weight and burn a high amount of fat.

As you start to get muscle, the weight will begin to drop more slowly. This is not because your fat is deciding to stick around but because muscle just weighs more than fat.

Even if your scale begins to slow down, your waistline is going to continue to shrink.

So, as you are tracking your progress, remember to measure your waist as well as recording your weight so you can keep a more accurate measure of your progress.

Day 1	Habit #1
Day 2	Habit #1
Day 3	Habit #1
Day 4	Habit #1 Habit #2
Day 5	Habit #1 Habit #2
Day 6	Habit #1 Habit #2
Day 7	Habit #1 Habit #2 Habit #3
Day 8	Habit #1 Habit #2 Habit #3
Day 9	Habit #1 Habit #2 Habit #3
Day 10	Habit #1 Habit #2 Habit #3 Habit #4
Day 11	Habit #1 Habit #2 Habit #3 Habit #4
Day 12	Habit #1 Habit #2 Habit #3 Habit #4
Day 13	Habit #1 Habit #2 Habit #3 Habit #4 Habit #5
Day 14	Habit #1 Habit #2 Habit #3 Habit #4 Habit #5
Day 15	Habit #1 Habit #2 Habit #3 Habit #4 Habit #5
Day 16	Habit #1 Habit #2 Habit #3 Habit #4 Habit #5 Habit #6
Day 17	Habit #1 Habit #2 Habit #3 Habit #4 Habit #5 Habit #6

Day 18	Habit #1 Habit #2 Habit #3 Habit #4 Habit #5 Habit #6
Day 19	Habit #1 Habit #2 Habit #3 Habit #4 Habit #5 Habit #6 Habit #7
Day 20	Habit #1 Habit #2 Habit #3 Habit #4 Habit #5 Habit #6 Habit #7
Day 21	Habit #1 Habit #2 Habit #3 Habit #4 Habit #5 Habit #6 Habit #7
Day 22	Habit #1 Habit #2 Habit #3 Habit #4 Habit #5 Habit #6 Habit #7 Habit #8
Day 23	Habit #1 Habit #2 Habit #3 Habit #4 Habit #5 Habit #6 Habit #7 Habit #8
Day 24	Habit #1 Habit #2 Habit #3 Habit #4 Habit #5 Habit #6 Habit #7 Habit #8
Day 25	Habit #1 Habit #2 Habit #3 Habit #4 Habit #5 Habit #6 Habit #7 Habit #8 Habit #9
Day 26	Habit #1 Habit #2 Habit #3 Habit #4 Habit #5 Habit #6 Habit #7 Habit #8 Habit #9
Day 27	Habit #1 Habit #2 Habit #3 Habit #4 Habit #5 Habit #6 Habit #7 Habit #8 Habit #9
Day 28	Habit #1 Habit #2 Habit #3 Habit #4 Habit #5 Habit #6 Habit #7 Habit #8 Habit #9 Habit #10
Day 29	Habit #1 Habit #2 Habit #3 Habit #4 Habit #5 Habit #6 Habit #7 Habit #8 Habit #9 Habit #10
Day 30	Habit #1 Habit #2 Habit #3 Habit #4 Habit #5 Habit #6 Habit #7 Habit #8 Habit #9 Habit #10

Continue adding one habit every fourth day for the next 30 days as well and you will have all 20 healthy evening habits established.

By the third month, they will become so engrained that you will hardly have to think about doing them.

They will just come naturally and be part of your new lifestyle that will help you lose weight and be healthier overall.

Conclusion

You have now read through all 21 healthy evening habits that can help you stick to a healthy diet and lose weight faster.

The final habit (doing the 30-day challenge) will help you stay on track and stay motivated to adopt the other 20 habits.

Remember to take it a step at a time and track your progress.

Achieving goals is just as much about appreciating how far you've come as it is about focusing on how far you have left to go.

It is also important to be prepared to make mistakes. The biggest and most worthwhile changes you make in your life don't come easily and they don't happen all at once.

If you could perfectly adopt a new, healthy habit without making a single mistake or slip up, which would mean it was already a habit of yours to begin with.

So be prepared for slip ups and don't let them bring you down and stop your progress. There will be days where it feels frustrating and difficult. You will want to give up.

But these are exactly the days that will make you stronger. For each tough day you push through and each slip you get back up from, you will be that much stronger and that much closer to achieving your weight loss goals.

The stronger you get, the easier it will be to get through the next tough day.

Your mistakes are not a sign of weakness. They are a sign that you are challenging yourself to do better. It's like exercise. If you've really pushed yourself during a workout, you're going to have sore muscles because the exercise has actually torn them.

It's the process of repairing those tears that makes you grow stronger.

So, remember: it's the process of making mistakes and pushing past them that will give you the strength and will power you need to achieve your goals.

Start practicing your new, healthy evening habits today and take pride in each step you take along the way!

Final Words

I would like to thank you for downloading my book and I hope I have been able to help you and educate you about something new.

If you have enjoyed this book and would like to share your positive thoughts, could you please take 30 seconds of your time to go back and give me a review on my Amazon book page!

I greatly appreciate seeing these reviews because it helps me share my hard work!

Again, thank you and I wish you all the best with your weight loss journey!

Disclaimer

This book and related sites provide wellness management information in an informative and educational manner only, with information that is general in nature and that is not specific to you, the reader. The contents of this site are intended to assist you and other readers in your personal wellness efforts. Consult your physician regarding the applicability of any information provided in our sites to you.

Nothing in this book should be construed as personal advices or diagnosis, and must not be used in this manner. The information provided about conditions is general in nature. This information does not cover all possible uses, actions, precautions, side-effects, or interactions of medicines, or medical procedures. The information in this site should not be considered as complete and does not cover all diseases, ailments, physical conditions, or their treatment.

You should **consult with your physician before beginning any exercise, weight loss, or healthcare program**. This book **should not** be used in place of a call or visit to a competent health-care professional. You should consult a health care professional before adopting any of the suggestions in this book or before drawing inferences from it.

Any decision regarding treatment and medication for your condition should be made with the advice and consultation of a qualified health care professional. If you have, or suspect you have, a health-care problem, then you should immediately contact a qualified health care professional for treatment.

No Warranties: The authors and publishers don't guarantee or warrant the quality, accuracy, completeness, timeliness, appropriateness or suitability of the information in this book, or of any product or services referenced by this site.

The information in this site is provided on an "as is" basis and the authors and publishers make no representations or warranties of any kind with respect to this information. This site may contain inaccuracies, typographical errors, or other errors.

Liability Disclaimer: The publishers, authors, and other parties involved in the creation, production, provision of information, or delivery of this site specifically disclaim any responsibility, and shall not be held liable for any damages, claims, injuries, losses, liabilities, costs, or obligations including any direct, indirect, special, incidental, or consequences damages (collectively known as "Damages") whatsoever and howsoever caused, arising out of, or in connection with the use or misuse of the site and the information contained within it, whether such Damages arise in contract, tort, negligence, equity, statute law, or by way of other legal theory.

37917109R00076

Made in the USA
Middletown, DE
03 March 2019